Osteoporosis Diet

A Beginner's Step-by-Step Guide To Preventing and Reversing Osteoporosis Through Nutrition With Recipes and a Meal Plan

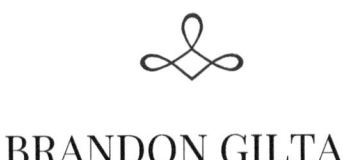

BRANDON GILTA

All rights reserved No part of this book may be reproduced, or stored in a retrieval system, or transmitted in any form or by any means, electronic, mechanical, photocopying, recording, or otherwise, without express written permission of the publisher.

Copyright © 2019 Brandon Gilta

All rights reserved.

Disclaimer

By reading this disclaimer, you are accepting the terms of the disclaimer in full. If you disagree with this disclaimer, please do not read the guide.

All of the content within this guide is provided for informational and educational purposes only, and should not be accepted as independent medical or other professional advice. The author is not a doctor, physician, nurse, mental health provider, or registered nutritionist/dietician. Therefore, using and reading this guide does not establish any form of a physician-patient relationship.

Always consult with a physician or another qualified health provider with any issues or questions you might have regarding any sort of medical condition. Do not ever disregard any qualified professional medical advice or delay seeking that advice because of anything you have read in this guide. The information in this guide is not intended to be any sort of medical advice and should not be used in lieu of any medical advice by a licensed and qualified medical professional.

The information in this guide has been compiled from a variety of known sources. However, the author cannot attest to or guarantee the accuracy of each source and thus should not be held liable for any errors or omissions.

You acknowledge that the publisher of this guide will not be held liable for any loss or damage of any kind incurred as a result of this guide or the reliance on any information provided within this guide. You acknowledge and agree that you assume all risk and responsibility for any action you undertake in response to the information in this guide.

Using this guide does not guarantee any particular result (e.g., weight loss or a cure). By reading this guide, you acknowledge that there are no guarantees to any specific outcome or results you can expect.

All product names, diet plans, or names used in this guide are for identification purposes only and are the property of their respective owners. The use of these names does not imply endorsement. All other trademarks cited herein are the property of their respective owners.

Where applicable, this guide is not intended to be a substitute for the original work of this diet plan and is, at most, a supplement to the original work for this diet plan and never a direct substitute. This guide is a personal expression of the facts of that diet plan.

Where applicable, persons shown in the cover images are stock photography models and the publisher has obtained the rights to use the images through license agreements with third-party stock image companies.

Introduction

Are you aware of the bony truth about osteoporosis? This disease may not be as well-known as cancer or heart disease, but it can have a significant impact on your health and overall quality of life. Osteoporosis is a condition that weakens bones, making them fragile and more susceptible to fractures. It's often referred to as the "silent disease" because it can progress undetected for years until a fracture occurs.

The good news is that there are steps you can take to help prevent osteoporosis and maintain strong bones. One of the most effective ways to do this is through diet. A healthy diet rich in calcium and vitamin D can help keep bones strong and reduce the risk of fractures.

Calcium is essential for building and maintaining strong bones. You should aim to consume at least 1,000 milligrams of calcium per day if you're under 50 years old, and 1,200 milligrams per day if you're over 50. Good sources of calcium include dairy products like milk, cheese, and yogurt, as well as leafy green vegetables like kale and broccoli.

Vitamin D is also important for bone health because it helps your body absorb calcium. You can get vitamin D from sunlight exposure or by consuming foods like fatty fish (such as salmon), egg yolks, and fortified cereals.

In addition to these nutrients, a diet rich in fruits, vegetables, whole grains, lean protein sources (like chicken or fish), and healthy fats (like olive oil) can also help promote overall health and reduce the risk of chronic diseases like heart disease and diabetes.

Remember that prevention is key when it comes to osteoporosis. By incorporating these dietary changes into your lifestyle early on, you can help maintain strong bones and reduce your risk of fractures later in life. Stay tuned for more tips on how to prevent osteoporosis through nutrition!

In this guide, we'll explore the following topics about osteoporosis and osteoporosis diet:

- Signs of osteoporosis
- Causes of osteoporosis
- How to prevent osteoporosis
- The principles of the osteoporosis diet
- A weekly guide for osteoporosis diet

So, let's dive in and get started!

Table of Contents

What Is Osteoporosis? 1
Causes and Risk Factors of Osteoporosis 7
Preventions and Treatments for Osteoporosis 11
The Principle of Osteoporosis Diet 15
Benefits of Osteoporosis Diet 17
Week 1: Learning about Osteoporosis 19
Week 2: Meal Plan Preparation 22
Week 3: Managing Osteoporosis 35
Sample Recipes 37

WHAT IS OSTEOPOROSIS?

Osteoporosis, which translates to "porous bones," is a type of disease that reduces the quality and density of the bones. As the bones turn porous, it becomes more fragile, increasing the risk of fracture. Bone loss happens progressively and silently and symptoms often, symptoms manifest at the first fracture.

Osteoporosis is common among women aged 50 and older, although there are cases where younger women are affected. Women are more prone to osteoporosis due to the reduction of estrogen levels. When a woman hits the menopausal stage, estrogen production greatly drops resulting in the osteoblast's inability to produce bones effectively.

Signs of Osteoporosis

There are no signs that would tell you are suffering from osteoporosis at least until the first fracture occurs. However, once it happens, you might notice the following signs:

Back pain or a hunched posture – A major indicator of osteoporosis is back pain or a hunched posture. If you're experiencing this symptom, it's important to understand the causes, so you can take appropriate steps to protect your bone health.

As your bones weaken over time, they become more susceptible to compression fractures in your spine. These fractures can cause you to experience back pain that may limit your mobility and daily activities. To identify the reason for your pain, a doctor may recommend a bone density scan or X-ray, as these tests can help diagnose osteoporosis and detect any existing fractures.

A hunched posture, also known as kyphosis or a "dowager's hump," is another sign of osteoporosis. It results from multiple compression fractures in your spine, causing the vertebrae to collapse and alter the shape of your spine. This change in alignment forces you to bend forward, leading to a hunched and stooped appearance.

Loss of height – Osteoporosis, a condition that weakens your bones, can have a subtle but noticeable impact on your life: a loss of height. This might happen as the vertebrae in your spine begin to compress or collapse due to the thinning of your bones. Over time, these changes can add up and cause you to become shorter than you once were. Pay attention to this shift, as it could be an important sign that you need to take action to safeguard your bone health.

Fractures – As someone potentially facing osteoporosis, you should be aware of the increased risk of fractures that comes with this condition. Osteoporosis causes a weakening in bone density, making them more susceptible to breaking even from minor injuries. This fragility is particularly dangerous for crucial areas like your hips, wrists, and spine.

Take extra care in your everyday activities to avoid accidents that could result in these fractures. Hip fractures can severely impact mobility and independence, while wrist fractures might hinder your ability to perform basic tasks. Spinal fractures, on the other hand, can lead to chronic pain and a decreased quality of life. Make it a priority to monitor your bone health and take steps to prevent osteoporosis-related fractures.

Weak grip strength – If you are having difficulty with grip strength, it may be a sign of osteoporosis. Your hands may feel weaker when trying to open jars or do other common tasks that require grip strength. Osteoporosis is a condition where strong bones become weak and brittle due to a lack of minerals such as calcium or vitamin D. This disease can cause bones to become easily fractured or broken, especially in the spine, hip, and wrist. Low bone density is often the main indicator of osteoporosis, but if not detected early on, weak grip strength can be another sign of this disease.

Brittle nails – When examining your nails, be aware that their condition can provide valuable insight into your overall bone health. If you consistently notice that your nails are weak and brittle, breaking easily, this may be an early indicator of osteoporosis. The structure and substances that make up your nails, such as collagen and minerals, are closely related to the components of your bones.

A decline in nail health can signify a decline in bone density and strength, putting you at greater risk for fractures and other osteoporosis-related issues. By paying close attention to this seemingly small detail, you might be able to recognize a potential problem and take the necessary steps to prevent or manage osteoporosis.

Receding gums or loose teeth – If you notice your gums receding or your teeth feeling loose, it could be a sign of osteoporosis affecting your jawbone. As your bone density decreases, the jawbone that supports your teeth may become weaker and less able to hold them securely in place. This can result in a shrinking gum line or teeth that start to wobble. In some cases, tooth loss may even occur.

To determine if osteoporosis is causing these symptoms, consult with your dentist and healthcare provider. They may recommend bone density tests or additional examinations to better understand your oral health and bone strength. Don't ignore these warning signs; addressing osteoporosis early can help prevent further bone deterioration and improve your overall health.

Stooped posture – If you notice a stooped posture developing, it might be a sign of osteoporosis progression. As your bones weaken and vertebral fractures become more frequent, your spine may start to curve forward, leading to an unmistakable hunched appearance known as kyphosis. This postural change not only affects your appearance but also contributes to the severity of the condition. It can result in difficulties with breathing, digestion, and even mobility, as your body struggles to adapt to the shifting bone structure.

To identify this sign early on and intervene effectively, pay close attention to any changes in your posture and consult a healthcare professional if you suspect osteoporosis is the cause. Understanding this critical sign can help you take proactive steps in managing your bone health and reducing the risks associated with osteoporosis.

Bone pain – If you're experiencing persistent bone pain, it could be a sign of osteoporosis. This debilitating condition often targets areas such as your hips, wrists, or spine, causing discomfort and negatively impacting your daily life. It's essential to pay close attention to these painful sensations, as osteoporosis weakens your bones, leaving them more susceptible to fractures.

Early detection can make a significant difference in managing the condition and improving your quality of life. So, don't ignore that ache, visit your doctor to discuss your symptoms and explore potential treatment options. Remember, with osteoporosis, being proactive about your bone health can help you maintain a strong, pain-free foundation for years to come.

Difficulty standing or walking – As you age, it's crucial to be aware of potential signs of osteoporosis, especially as it may severely affect your overall mobility. One significant warning sign to look out for is experiencing difficulty standing or walking without assistance. This challenge typically arises from fractures caused by the weakening of your bones due to osteoporosis. Such fractures may not only exacerbate existing mobility issues but can also lead to severe pain and long-lasting complications. If you notice increased difficulty in moving, it's essential to consult a healthcare professional to determine if osteoporosis is the underlying cause.

Frequent falls – If you're experiencing frequent falls, it may be an indicator that you have osteoporosis. This condition causes your bones to weaken, making you more susceptible to falls and fractures. As a result, even a minor stumble or slip may lead to serious injuries. When your bones lose density, they become fragile and break more easily—a hallmark sign of osteoporosis.

It's crucial to pay attention to this warning sign and consult your doctor for a comprehensive evaluation. They can determine if osteoporosis is the cause of your frequent falls and help design a personalized treatment plan to improve your bone health.

Prevention is the key to fighting osteoporosis. Do not wait for the signs or for the first fracture to occur. It's important to note that not everyone with osteoporosis will experience all of these symptoms. Additionally, some people may not experience any symptoms at all until they have a fracture. That's why it's important to talk to your doctor about your risk factors for osteoporosis and getting regular bone density screenings is recommended.

CAUSES AND RISK FACTORS OF OSTEOPOROSIS

Osteoporosis is a condition that affects millions of people worldwide, causing bones to become fragile and prone to fractures. While it's more common in older women, anyone can develop osteoporosis. There are several causes and risk factors that can contribute to the development of this condition, including:

Age – As you age, your bones naturally become less dense and weaker, increasing your risk of developing osteoporosis. This gradual weakening process occurs because the older bone is continuously broken down and replaced by new bone. However, as you get older, your body's ability to generate fresh bone to replace the old deteriorates, resulting in a net loss of bone mass. Consequently, your bones become more fragile and prone to fractures.

Gender – Osteoporosis, a degenerative bone disease, presents a higher risk for women than men, primarily due to hormonal changes women experience during menopause. Estrogen, a key hormone in maintaining bone strength and density, decreases significantly in postmenopausal women. This reduction in estrogen levels leads to an accelerated rate of bone loss and, consequently, a greater likelihood of developing osteoporosis.

Research indicates that women can lose up to 20% of their bone density within the first five to seven years following menopause, leaving them more vulnerable to fractures and serious complications. Approximately 80% of the individuals diagnosed with osteoporosis are female. Although men also experience age-related bone loss, their risk remains lower due to higher peak bone mass and a slower decline in bone density compared to women.

Efforts to mitigate postmenopausal osteoporosis in women include hormone replacement therapy, adequate calcium, and vitamin D intake, and engaging in regular weight-bearing activities, as these measures help maintain bone strength and reduce the risk of fractures.

Genetics – Genetic factors significantly influence an individual's susceptibility to osteoporosis. Specific genes regulate bone development, density, and remodel process, thereby determining a person's predisposition to this debilitating condition. Consequently, people with a family history of osteoporosis exhibit a higher risk of developing it themselves. Understanding one's genetic background enables one to take necessary preventive measures and maintain bone health throughout their life.

Lifestyle factors – Osteoporosis often develops due to various lifestyle factors. An absence of regular physical activity weakens bones, while smoking exacerbates bone loss. Excessive alcohol consumption interferes with the body's ability to absorb calcium, a vital mineral for bone health. Additionally, poor nutrition deprives bones of essential nutrients, accelerating the onset of osteoporosis. Maintaining a healthy lifestyle with exercise, proper nutrition, and moderate alcohol intake helps preserve bone density and prevent this debilitating condition.

Medical conditions – Numerous medical conditions contribute to an increased risk of osteoporosis. Thyroid disorders, specifically hyperthyroidism, cause bone loss by speeding up the body's natural bone replacement process. Inflammatory bowel disease disrupts nutrient absorption, leading to calcium deficiencies that hinder bone development. Additionally, eating disorders like anorexia nervosa may cause hormonal imbalances, resulting in decreased bone density and an increased risk of fractures.

Medications – Prolonged use of specific medications contributes to the onset of osteoporosis. Corticosteroids, taken for chronic conditions like asthma and rheumatoid arthritis, can weaken bone density over time. Additionally, anticonvulsants for epilepsy and aromatase inhibitors for breast cancer increase the likelihood of bone fragility. Monitoring medication effects vigilantly remains crucial in mitigating osteoporosis risks.

Body size – A small body frame or low body weight significantly increases one's risk of developing osteoporosis. This heightened vulnerability occurs because thinner individuals possess less bone mass, providing a weaker foundation. As bones naturally weaken with age, those with a smaller frame or lower body weight face a greater likelihood of experiencing fragility fractures and osteoporosis-related complications. It's crucial for people in this category to engage in activities that can help increase bone mass to mitigate the risk.

Hormonal imbalances – Osteoporosis often results from hormonal imbalances, specifically when men experience low testosterone levels or when individuals have excessive thyroid hormone production. These imbalances can lead to a decline in bone density, leaving bones more fragile and susceptible to fractures. Maintaining proper hormonal levels is crucial for preserving bone strength and overall health.

Previous fractures – A history of previous fractures significantly increases the risk of osteoporosis. Weakened bones, resulting from prior fractures, make individuals more susceptible to future bone breaks. This heightened vulnerability may also exacerbate existing bone loss, further compromising one's bone health. Therefore, it is crucial for those with a fracture history to seek medical advice and take preventative measures, to ensure their bones remain strong and healthy.

It's important to understand that while some risk factors for osteoporosis cannot be controlled (such as age and genetics), there are several lifestyle changes you can make to reduce your risk of developing this condition.

PREVENTIONS AND TREATMENTS FOR OSTEOPOROSIS

There are many preventions and treatments available to manage symptoms and reduce the risk of fractures. These include:

1. Exercise regularly

To prevent osteoporosis, individuals must engage in consistent, targeted physical activities. Weight-bearing exercises such as walking, jogging, and dancing promote overall bone strength, while resistance training, including weightlifting and resistance bands, specifically targets the spine and other vulnerable areas. By adopting a proactive exercise routine, individuals can effectively minimize their risk of developing osteoporosis and maintain strong, healthy bones throughout their lifetime.

2. Get enough calcium and vitamin D

Incorporating calcium and vitamin D into a daily routine significantly impacts osteoporosis prevention. Both nutrients form an essential partnership - calcium strengthens the bone structure, while vitamin D bolsters calcium absorption. To maintain optimum bone health, individuals must consume calcium-rich foods or supplements and ensure consistent exposure to sunlight for optimal vitamin D synthesis. Prioritizing these actions helps counteract osteoporosis development, leading to a lower risk of fractures and increased overall wellness.

3. Avoid smoking and excessive alcohol consumption

To prevent osteoporosis, individuals should abstain from smoking and limit alcohol intake, as these habits can harm bone health. Smoking decreases bone density, while excessive alcohol consumption disrupts the body's calcium absorption and balance. For optimal bone strength, it is crucial to adopt a healthy lifestyle that involves making informed choices regarding smoking and alcohol consumption.

4. Take medications as prescribed

To effectively prevent osteoporosis, individuals should consistently take prescribed medications as directed by their healthcare provider. These drugs slow down bone loss and promote the formation of new bone, ultimately strengthening and preserving the skeletal system. Proper adherence to suggested medical treatments is vital to mitigate osteoporosis' consequences and maintain optimal bone health.

5. Eat a balanced diet

To prevent osteoporosis, individuals should maintain a balanced diet containing essential nutrients for bone health. This involves consuming fruits, vegetables, whole grains, lean proteins, and healthy fats. Such nutrient-rich foods contribute to the development of strong bones, thereby reducing the risk of osteoporosis and promoting overall skeletal health.

6. Maintain a healthy weight

Maintaining an optimal weight significantly reduces the risk of osteoporosis development. Underweight individuals face a higher susceptibility due to insufficient bone density, while excessive weight can lead to weakened bone structure. Ensuring a well-balanced diet and regular exercise helps achieve a healthy weight, promoting strong bones and preventing the onset of osteoporosis.

7. Reduce your risk of falls

Preventing osteoporosis involves minimizing the risk of falls, as these incidents can result in serious fractures. To enhance safety, individuals should prioritize wearing suitable footwear with proper support, maintaining a clutter-free home environment with adequate lighting, and utilizing beneficial assistive devices when necessary.

8. Get regular bone density tests

Bone density tests can help detect osteoporosis early on before any symptoms occur. Your doctor may recommend a bone density test if you are at high risk for osteoporosis.

9. Consider hormone replacement therapy (HRT)

HRT may be recommended for postmenopausal women to help prevent bone loss and reduce the risk of fractures.

10. Participate in fall prevention programs

Some community centers offer fall prevention programs that include exercises to improve balance and coordination, as well as education on how to prevent falls.

As for cures, there is currently no cure for osteoporosis. However, treatments are available to manage symptoms and slow down bone loss. Your doctor may prescribe medications such as bisphosphonates or hormone therapy to help prevent fractures and improve bone density.

Remember to always consult with your healthcare provider before starting any new exercise routine or treatment plan for osteoporosis.

THE PRINCIPLE OF OSTEOPOROSIS DIET

When it comes to preventing or managing osteoporosis, diet is an important factor. A balanced diet rich in vitamins, minerals, and nutrients can help support bone health and reduce the risk of fractures and other complications associated with this condition. Here are some general dietary principles that may help:

1. **Consume adequate amounts of calcium** – Adequate calcium intake is essential for building and maintaining strong bones. The recommended daily amount of calcium for adults aged 19-50 is 1000 mg/day, while those over 50 should aim for 1200 mg/day. Good sources of calcium include dairy products, dark green leafy vegetables, salmon, sardines, and fortified foods like orange juice and cereals.
2. **Get enough vitamin D** – Vitamin D is needed to absorb calcium and promote bone health. The recommended daily amount of vitamin D for adults aged 19-70 is 600 IU/day, while those over 70 should aim for 800 IU/day. Food sources of vitamin D include fatty fish, egg yolks, fortified milk, and some mushrooms.
3. **Increase the consumption of fruits and vegetables** – Fruits and vegetables are rich in vitamins and minerals

that can help support bone health. Aim to include at least 5 servings of fruits and vegetables in your daily diet.
4. **Eat foods high in protein** – Protein helps build and maintain muscle mass which can help reduce the risk of falls and fractures. Good sources of protein include lean meats, poultry, fish, eggs, legumes, nuts, and seeds.
5. **Limit sodium intake** – High sodium intake can increase calcium excretion in the urine and weaken bones over time. Try to limit your daily salt intake to 2,300 mg or less per day.
6. **Limit caffeine consumption** – Caffeine can interfere with the absorption of calcium, so it's important to limit the consumption of coffee, tea, and other caffeinated beverages.
7. **Avoid processed foods and added sugars** – Processed foods are often high in sodium and added sugars which can weaken bones over time. Try to limit your consumption of processed and sugary foods, and opt for whole, nutrient-rich foods instead.

By following these dietary guidelines, you can take an active role in protecting your bone health and reducing the risk of osteoporosis-related fractures. However, it's important to remember that diet alone is not enough to prevent or treat osteoporosis. You should also be getting adequate amounts of exercise and regular check-ups with your healthcare provider. Taking these steps can help ensure you maintain strong bones for years to come!

BENEFITS OF OSTEOPOROSIS DIET

Here are some of the benefits one can reap by following an osteoporosis diet:

Reduces the Risk of Fractures – One of the primary benefits of an osteoporosis diet is that it can help to reduce the risk of fractures. Osteoporosis is a condition that causes bones to become weak and brittle, and as a result, even a minor fall can lead to a fracture. A diet that is rich in calcium and vitamin D can help to strengthen bones and reduce the risk of fractures.

Improves Bone density – Another benefit of an osteoporosis diet is that it can improve bone density. Bone density is a measure of how much bone tissue is present in a given area. A diet that is rich in calcium and vitamin D can help to increase bone density and reduce the risk of osteoporosis.

Reduces Inflammation – An osteoporosis diet can also help to reduce inflammation. Inflammation is a natural process that occurs when the body's immune system responds to an injury or infection. However, chronic inflammation can lead to a variety of health problems, including osteoporosis. A diet that includes anti-inflammatory foods such as omega-3 fatty acids can help to reduce inflammation and protect against osteoporosis.

Lowers Blood Pressure – An osteoporosis diet can also help to lower blood pressure. High blood pressure puts extra strain on the arteries and bones, which can lead to fractures. A diet that is low in salt and fat can help to lower blood pressure and reduce the risk of osteoporosis.

Improves Kidney Function – An osteoporosis diet can also help to improve kidney function. Kidneys play an important role in regulating calcium levels in the body, and a diet that is rich in calcium can help to improve kidney function and reduce the risk of osteoporosis.

Increases Muscle Mass – An osteoporosis diet can also help to increase muscle mass. Muscle mass helps to support bones and reduces the likelihood of fractures. A diet that includes protein-rich foods such as meat, poultry, fish, tofu, and beans can help to increase muscle mass and reduce the risk of osteoporosis.

Reduces Body Fat Percentage – An osteoporosis diet can also help to reduce body fat percentage. Excess body fat puts extra strain on bones and increases the likelihood of fractures. A diet that includes healthy fats such as olive oil, nuts, and avocados can help to reduce body fat percentage and protect against osteoporosis.

WEEK 1: LEARNING ABOUT OSTEOPOROSIS

Osteoporosis is not like a weight-loss problem where you can decide to start a new diet and your problem will be okay. You cannot just decide that you have osteoporosis and should start an Osteoporosis diet.

Step 1: Getting Tested

The first thing you need to do is get a bone density test. A bone density test will help you check how strong your bones are. Being tested does not mean you have the disease. You are merely taking the first and most important preventive measure against the disease. To determine if you need a bone density test you should fall under the following categories:

- You are over the age of 50
- You are female
- You are postmenopausal
- You are a male over 70 and have not had a bone density test
- You have a family history of the disease
- You have been taking steroids for far too long
- You have a medical condition like rheumatoid arthritis

- You smoke and drink

These are just a few reasons that would put you at a higher risk of the disease.

Step 2: Learning more about the disease

Once tested and you are found to have osteoporosis, talk to your doctor. Do not be afraid to ask questions. Learn more about the disease. Here are a few important things you need to learn:

- What is the gravity of your disease? Are you in the early stage or is your curvature already at an odd angle?
- How does osteoporosis affect your existing medical condition? (if you have any)
- What kind of treatment do you need?
- What do you need to do to reverse the disease? Can you still reverse the disease?
- What other complications should you expect with the disease?

Step 3: Changing your Lifestyle

The causes of osteoporosis are treatable, even lack of estrogen. Some women undergo Hormonal Replacement Therapy to combat the drop of estrogen at the onset of menopause but this is not a lifetime solution.

What you need is to change your lifestyle. If you smoke or drink, you have to reduce if not remove it from your habit. You also need to do exercises that are more physical and change your diet. You can make these changes under the guidance of your physician especially if you have a medical condition.

WEEK 2: MEAL PLAN PREPARATION

One of the biggest changes you need to undergo is the way you eat and what foods you eat. If you have osteoporosis, the most important nutrients your body needs are Vitamin D and Calcium.

Step 1: Determining what foods you need

If you are going on an Osteoporosis Diet, you will need foods rich in calcium and Vitamin D. The daily calcium intake depends partly on your gender and age:

- Children aged 0 – 9 = range from 300 to 700 milligrams daily
- Adolescents aged 10 to 18 = 1,300 milligrams daily
- Women 19 – menopausal stage = 1,000 milligrams daily
- Women postmenopausal stage = 1,300 milligrams daily
- Women in the last trimester of pregnancy = 1200 milligrams daily
- Women in lactation period = 1,000 milligrams daily
- Men 19 – 65 years = 1,000 milligrams daily

- Men 65 and over = 1,300 milligrams daily

For daily Vitamin D intake

- 0-9 years = 200 UI
- 10-18 years = 200 UI
- 19-50 years = 200 UI
- 51-65 years = 400 UI
- 65+ years = 600 UI
- Pregnancy = 200 UI
- Lactation = 200 UI

Consult with your physician to help you determine what daily calcium and Vitamin D intake you need and ask for a table of foods rich in calcium and vitamin D that you can eat.

Recommended Foods

Eating the right kinds of food can help to reduce the risk of Osteoporosis and its effects. Below is a list of 15 recommended foods that provide important minerals and vitamins for better bone health.

1. Leafy green vegetables:

Leafy green vegetables like kale, spinach, collard greens, and Swiss chard are rich in minerals such as calcium and magnesium. These minerals are important for bone health as they help to retain bone mass and reduce the risk of fractures associated with osteoporosis.

2. Dairy products:

Dairy products like milk, cheese, and yogurt contain high levels of calcium and vitamin D which are essential for strong bones. Calcium helps strengthen bones, while vitamin D aids in the absorption of calcium into the bones.

3. Tofu:

Tofu is a great source of plant-based protein and contains the same amount of calcium as cow's milk. It can be added to salads or stir-fries to increase your dietary intake of calcium.

4. Almonds:

Almonds are a great source of healthy fats, magnesium, phosphorus, zinc, and vitamins A and E which all play an important role in maintaining healthy bones and reducing the risk of fractures associated with osteoporosis.

5. Salmon:

Salmon is full of omega-3 fatty acids which help to reduce inflammation in the body that can contribute to weakened bones over time. Additionally, salmon also helps to balance hormones that affect bone strength in both menopausal women and aging men who are susceptible to osteoporosis.

6. Sesame seeds:

Sesame seeds are a powerful source of copper and zinc, both of which play an important role in protecting bones. Copper helps fend off free radical damage while zinc balances hormones that directly affect bone strength, making sesame seeds particularly beneficial for those at risk of developing osteoporosis.

7. Legumes:

Legumes such as chickpeas, lentils, and beans are a powerful source of essential minerals like zinc, magnesium, iron, and phosphorus that help promote strong bones throughout one's lifespan. Eating legumes daily can be an easy and delicious way to decrease the risk of developing osteoporosis.

8. Whole Grains:

Eating whole grains like barley, oats, and quinoa can provide your body with essential energy and strength to help you maintain good bone health. Whole grains regulate your blood sugar levels, providing a steady source of energy throughout the day to support your exercise sessions and improve your overall health.

9. Egg yolks:

Egg yolks are an excellent source of Vitamin D and Vitamin K, both of which have been found to have a positive impact on bone health. Vitamin D helps with calcium absorption, improving the strength and longevity of bones, while Vitamin K is essential for effective blood clotting and can help prevent injuries due to falls, making it a great choice for those suffering from osteoporosis.

10. Sunflower Seeds:

Sunflower seeds are packed with beneficial nutrients such as unsaturated fats, magnesium, and vitamins C and E that have been proven to help reduce the risk of developing osteoporosis. Vitamin C and E are strong antioxidants that help fight inflammation-related triggers associated with the condition, while magnesium and unsaturated fats increase bone density and help protect bones from further damage.

11. Avocados:

Avocados are a nutritious superfood packed with monounsaturated fats and Omega-3 fatty acids, which help to improve bone health and avoid the onset or progression of Osteoporosis. Vitamin B6 and Vitamin K found in avocados provide additional support to fortify bones and decrease stress, making it an ideal food choice for those looking to benefit their bone health.

12. Broccoli:

Broccoli has long been heralded as a powerhouse of nutrition, and it holds particular promise for individuals grappling with bone loss conditions. Rich in vitamins A, D, and C, these essential nutrients work in tandem to support proper utilization and digestion, fostering a healthy environment for our skeletal systems.

13. Oysters:

Oysters are a great source of zinc, which helps to regulate hormonal balance and minimize the risk of osteoporosis during menopause. Regular consumption of oysters can provide valuable nutrients that help support overall well-being during this time of transition.

14. Citrus Fruits:

The abundance of vitamin C found in citrus fruits, such as apples, oranges, and grapefruits, not only adds a refreshing zest to your diet but also plays a crucial role in combating free radical damage. Scientists have found that an ever-increasing influx of these unstable molecules can potentially contribute to a decline in bone mass buildup.

15. Peaches and nectarines:

The delectable taste of peaches and nectarines does more than just tantalize your taste buds; they also pack a nutritional punch that helps to bolster nerve transmission functions. This potent ability is particularly noteworthy for those experiencing moderate osteoporotic progression, which often leads to hampered mobility and restricted movements.

These are just a few examples of the many foods that can be incorporated into an osteoporosis diet guide to help reduce the risk of developing or exacerbating this debilitating condition. The key is to find a nutritious balance that works best for your needs and lifestyle while ensuring vitamin and mineral fortification throughout.

Foods to Avoid

If you suffer from osteoporosis, changing your diet to include healthy foods and avoiding certain ones can help reduce your risk of further bone loss and maintain better overall health. Here are 15 foods that should be avoided if you have osteoporosis and why.

1. **Carbonated drinks:** Carbonated drinks can cause the leaching of calcium from the bones, which can lead to a decrease in bone density and osteoporosis.
2. **Caffeinated drinks:** Caffeine can increase the excretion of calcium through urine, thus causing a decrease in bone density and osteoporosis.
3. **Refined grains:** Refined grains such as white bread, white rice, and pasta, lack essential vitamins and minerals needed for strong bones and can contribute to osteoporosis.
4. **Alcohol:** Alcohol has a direct effect on bone health by inhibiting bone formation and leading to bone loss which can increase the risk of osteoporosis.
5. **High-sodium foods:** High-sodium foods such as salty snacks, canned soups, processed meats, and fast food can lead to calcium excretion through urine, thus reducing bone mineral density and increasing the risk of osteoporosis.
6. **Processed meats:** Processed meats contain high levels of saturated fat which can lead to an increased risk of heart disease and stroke as well as an increased risk of developing osteoporosis due to decreased absorption of essential nutrients required for healthy bones.
7. **Excessive amounts of meat:** Eating more than one or two small servings a day can increase your chances of developing osteoporosis due to the high amount of animal protein contained within them that may interfere

with calcium absorption in the body leading to low bone density over time.
8. **Sugary foods/drinks:** These are typically low in essential vitamins and minerals that are essential for healthy bones such as calcium, magnesium, vitamin D and K—thus contributing to poor overall health that increases the risk of developing osteoporosis down the line.
9. **High-acidity foods/drinks (like soda):** Soda contains phosphoric acid, which can help to break down collagen fibers, a key structural component in bones. Consumption of acidic products leads to quicker breakdowns of materials, making it hard for us to replace these components when needed. This leads directly to weakened bones, such as those found in people with Osteoarthritis.
10. **High-fat dairy products:** When it comes to osteoarthritis management, it's crucial to understand the double-edged sword of high-fat dairy products. On one hand, they offer the beneficial calcium your body needs to maintain strong bones and overall health. However, the downside is the unhealthy saturated fat content, which can negatively impact those with osteoarthritis. Consuming these products can lead to an increase in cholesterol accumulation within the body, making it harder for you to effectively manage your weight—ultimately leading to weaker bones due to inflammation processes. Keep in mind that striking a balance in your diet will provide you with the required nutrients while mitigating the adverse effects of these dairy products.

By making simple changes to your diet and avoiding certain foods, you can help reduce the risk of further bone loss associated with osteoporosis.

Step 2 of Week 2: Making your Meal Plan

Once you know what type of foods to eat, you can make your meal plan. You can do this on your own or with the help of a Nutritionist. To start you off, here's a sample of a 7-day meal plan designed for people with Osteoporosis:

Day 1

Breakfast

- Orange juice fortified with Calcium and Vitamin D
- Cereal fortified with vitamin D, Whole grain
- 4 oz. the glass of skim milk

Lunch

- Oven-baked salmon with radish
- green salad with hard-boiled egg
- 8 oz. glass of skim milk

Snack

- 1 medium orange fruit

Dinner

- Grilled vermouth tuna
- 1/2 cup broccoli florets, steamed
- 3/4 cup brown rice
- 1 cup raspberries with lite whipped topping

Day 2

Breakfast

- 1 serving Oatmeal Yogurt Smoothie
- 4 oz. fortified orange juice

Lunch

- 1 serving of mushroom and onion brown risotto
- cucumber, avocado, and cherry tomato salad
- small serving of sorbet with raspberries

Snack

- • Greek yogurt with sliced fruit or berries

Dinner

- Whole grain Spaghetti pesto and feta
- falafel pita sandwich with cucumber, lettuce, and tomato
- 1 small serving of lemon sorbet garnished with raspberry sauce

Day 3

Breakfast

- Red pumpkin pudding
- 8 oz. calcium and Vitamin D-fortified orange juice

Lunch

- Steamed Basmati Rice Bowl w/ Broccoli and Tofu
- 1 slice watermelon

Snack

- 1 banana

Dinner

- Pesto Chicken Cauliflower Pasta and Salad Mix
- mashed sweet potato

Day 4

Breakfast

- Baked Egg Sardines Casserole
- 2 slices French bread
- 8 oz. glass of skim milk

Lunch

- Artichoke Linguine in Spinach Pesto
- 2 slices French bread

- 1 apple or banana

Snack

- banana smoothie Greek yogurt or skim milk

Dinner

- grilled chicken sautéed with mushrooms, zucchini, and asparagus
- corn on the cob

Day 5

Breakfast

- Red pumpkin pudding
- 4 oz. glass of soy milk
- 1 small banana

Lunch

- Brazilian-style Spinach Casserole
- Grilled eggplant panini
- Green mix salad with tomatoes and basil

Snack

- chickpea bean dip
- 1 toasted whole-grain pita, sliced into fours for dipping

Dinner

- Ravioli in three cheese
- 2 slices French bread
- small serving sorbet with berry sauce or fruits

WEEK 3: MANAGING OSTEOPOROSIS

Once you have started treatment for Osteoporosis, the next hard step is managing it. Even if you are getting treatment or eating the right diet, slacking will not help you manage it.

Step 1: Adapting to your new Meal Plan

It is going to be an uphill battle. You will not only deal with the physical pain and possible side effects of medication (if you are advised to take medication), but you will also need to adapt to your new diet. Although meat, fish, and vegetables will be a big part of your diet, they will still be difficult to maintain. You need to remember that you are filling up your calcium and vitamin D deficiency.

This is not like a fad diet where you can have cheat days. This is unlike any other diet where you can skip a day and tell yourself, I'll start again tomorrow. If you skip or you stop, it can hurt your overall health. You need to remember that you are treating a disease.

Step 2: Creating habits to manage osteoporosis

Changing your lifestyle means changing old bad habits and creating new ones. If you drink and smoke, you need to eliminate it because alcohol and cigarettes lead to osteoporosis.

You also need to do some physical exercises to combat the sedentary condition of your bones and muscles. You can do brisk walking, jogging, dancing, aerobics, hiking, and other simple exercises. Again, be reminded that you need to clear all these habits with your physician.

Step 3: Regular Consultation with your physician

The last step is to maintain regular check-ups with your doctor. Osteoporosis is a chronic disease and you cannot treat it on your own. Consulting with your doctor will help you check on your progress and make necessary changes to your treatment.

SAMPLE RECIPES

Brazilian Style Spinach Casserole

Ingredients:

- 60 g vegetable oil non-stick spray
- 340 g spinach, frozen and thawed
- 475 g cooked brown rice
- 2 tbsp. olive oil
- 240 ml egg whites
- 65 g shredded mozzarella cheese
- 240 ml low-fat milk
- 1/2 medium chopped onion
- 1/4 tsp. oregano
- 1/4 tsp. dried thyme
- 1/4 tsp. dried rosemary
- 1/2 tsp. Worcestershire sauce

Instructions:

1. Prepare a large baking dish and spray with non-stick vegetable oil. Preheat the oven to 180°C.
2. Thaw the frozen spinach in a colander and press it to squeeze out excess water.

3. Place the drained spinach in a large mixing bowl.
4. Add in spices, milk, brown rice, egg whites, olive oil, cheese, and Worcestershire sauce. Mix until well combined.
5. Transfer the combined mixture to the prepared baking dish.
6. Place it in the oven and bake for 30 minutes.
7. Serve hot.

Steamed Basmati Rice Bowl with Broccoli and Tofu

Ingredients:

- 500 g tofu, firm, and low fat
- 2 cups basmati rice
- 2 whole broccoli florets
- 1/2 cup vegetable broth
- 2 tbsp. soya sauce, low salt
- 1 tbsp. black beans sauce
- 1-inch size ginger, minced
- 5 cloves garlic, minced
- 2 tbsp. brown sugar
- 1/2 tbsp. chili flakes
- Optional: 1 tbsp. dry sherry

Instructions:

1. Steam the basmati rice then set it aside.
2. Use a large shallow pan and combine the vegetable broth, soya sauce, black beans sauce, dry sherry

(optional), ginger, garlic, brown sugar, and chili flakes. Bring it to a boil.
3. Drain the tofu using kitchen towels and then cut it into 0.5-x-0.5-inch pieces.
4. Lather your tofu by turning it into broth.
5. Remove the tofu. Place a rack an inch high from the broth. Gently place the pieces of tofu onto the rack.
6. Cover the pan with foil then steam for 10 minutes on high heat. Remove the tofu after 10 minutes.
7. Add water to your boiling broth to raise it another inch deep then toss in the broccoli.
8. Let it cook for 4 minutes or until the broccoli turns tender.
9. Take a bowl of rice and spoon in some of the broth, and top with broccoli and tofu. Add soya sauce to taste.
10. Serve hot.

Ravioli in Three Cheese

Ingredients:

- 2 tsp. olive oil
- 3 tbsp. shallot, minced
- 1 bunch of red Swiss chard, trimmed and coarsely chopped
- 1/2 tsp. pepper, divided
- 3/4 cup part-skim ricotta cheese
- 1/2 cup fresh goat cheese
- 1/2 cup grated Parmesan cheese
- 1 tbsp. fresh sage, finely chopped
- 72 fresh or frozen square wonton wrappers, thawed

- 1/4 cup + 2 tbsp. store-bought pesto
- Optional: 6 small fresh sage leaves

Instructions

1. In a new bowl, combine all the cheese, chopped sage, and remaining pepper and mix well.
2. Layout a baking sheet lined with parchment paper and then lay out half of the wonton wrappers on the lined baking sheet.
3. Spoon 2 tsp. of the cheese mixture at the center of each wonton.
4. Dip the tip of your fingers in water and wet the edges of each wrapper.
5. Place another wrapper over the cheese filling and press down gently to seal the edges of the wonton then cover with plastic wrap and refrigerate for 1 day.
6. In a non-stick skillet, warm the oil over medium-low heat. Add the shallots and cook and stir for a minute.
7. Add the chard and half of the pepper and stir-cook for 3 minutes or until the leaves turn wilted.
8. Transfer the chard to a bowl to set aside but keep it warm.
9. In a large pot, bring to a boil a pot of salted water; reduce to a simmer.
10. Drop the prepared ravioli into the water; stir gently to prevent sticking. Let it simmer for 5 minutes.
11. Remove the ravioli using a slotted spoon and place them on paper towels to blot dry.
12. Arrange six ravioli in 6 bowls. Drizzle about 1 tbsp. of pesto over each bowl of ravioli.

13. Divide the cooked chard to fill six bowls. Garnish with sage, if you desire before serving.

Baked Egg Sardines Casserole

Ingredients:

- 1 125-g tin of sardines
- 4 eggs
- A handful of parsley, finely chopped
- 3 tbsp. finely diced shallot
- 2 cloves finely chopped garlic
- pepper
- salt

Instructions:

1. Turn the oven to 250°C and preheat an oven proof casserole for a few minutes.
2. Pour the sardines into the warm casserole dish; breaking them slightly apart with a fork.
3. Add the parsley, shallots, garlic, and ground black pepper.
4. Return the casserole dish to the oven and bake for 5 to 6 minutes, then remove from the oven.
5. Break four eggs on top of the baked sardines, arranging the eggs evenly spaced around the dish. Season with salt and pepper.
6. Return the casserole to the oven and bake for another 7 minutes or until egg whites are half-cooked and still wobbly.

7. Remove from the oven and let it sit for 5 minutes. The eggs will continue to cook while cooling.
8. Serve with toast or as a side dish to a salad. You can also enjoy it as is.

Mushroom and Onion Brown Risotto

Ingredients:

- 1 yellow or sweet onion, thinly sliced
- 2 tbsp. vegetable oil
- 450 g sliced mushrooms
- 190 g brown rice
- 60 ml dry white wine
- 480 ml vegetable broth
- 240 ml of water
- 225 g frozen peas
- 25 g Parmesan cheese, grated

Instructions

1. On a non-stick frying pan over medium heat, warm 1 tbsp. of oil.
2. Add onions and stir-cook for 3 minutes or until brown but not burnt. Remove from the pan and set aside.
3. Wipe the pan clean and heat the remaining oil.
4. Add the mushroom and cook for 15 minutes or until brown.
5. While browning the mushroom, cook the risotto by heating wine and brown rice in a pot. Stir until the rice absorbs the wine.

6. Add half of the broth and water and increase the heat to medium-high. Do not cover the pot and stir frequently until all liquid is absorbed.
7. Add the remaining liquid one cup at a time to allow each cup to be absorbed.
8. Add the peas with the last cup of liquid, and let the rice cook for an hour or until it turns tender and creamy.
9. Remove from heat. Gently stir in the browned onion and mushrooms.
10. Fold in the cheese and wait five minutes before serving.

Whole Grain Spaghetti in Pesto and Feta

Ingredients:

- 450 g spaghetti, whole grain
- 1 package (280 g) frozen spinach, thawed and well-drained
- 2 tbsp. olive oil
- 280 g frozen spinach, thawed
- 25 g shredded Parmesan cheese
- 2 cloves garlic
- 2 tbsp. melted butter
- 2 tbsp. chopped parsley
- 1/2 tsp. dried basil
- 1/2 tsp. salt
- 60 g feta cheese (crumbled)
- 80 ml of water

Instructions:

1. Prepare the pesto by mixing in the blender the oil, spinach, parmesan cheese, garlic, parsley, basil, and salt.
2. Blend the mixture until it turns into a fine mixture.
3. Add the melted butter gradually until blended.
4. Cook your pasta according to package instructions.
5. Toss the pesto mixture with the cooked pasta.
6. Top with crumbled feta cheese before serving.

Artichoke Linguine in Spinach Pesto

Ingredients:

- 1 large jar of artichoke hearts
- 250 g baby spinach
- 1 cup fresh basil
- 1/4 cup hemp hearts
- 1/2 cup nutritional yeast
- 1/4 cup pine nuts
- 1/2 red onion
- 1 tsp. black pepper
- 1 tbsp. lemon juice
- 1 tbsp. salt
- 1 tbsp. garlic
- 1 tbsp. apple cider
- A handful of fresh rocket
- 500 g linguine pasta

Instructions:

1. Chop onions and basil roughly then put in a food processor.
2. Add the artichoke hearts with a little of the artichoke oil preserved.
3. Add in the lemon juice, apple cider, hemp hearts, pepper, garlic, yeast, and half of the pine nuts.
4. Pulse several times until it turns smooth. Toss in the spinach and pulse again.
5. Add water if needed, until you get a smooth and creamy consistency.
6. Boil your pasta for 10 to 12 minutes or until al dente. Drain.
7. Simmer the pesto on medium heat and add in the remaining pine nuts and fresh rocket leaves.
8. Toss the pasta in and mix.
9. Serve and enjoy

Red Pumpkin Pudding

Ingredients:

1. 400 g red pumpkin
2. 1 tsp. cornflour
3. 200 ml of milk
4. 1/2 tbsp. cinnamon powder
5. 1 tsp. desiccated coconut
6. 1 tsp. pomegranate pearls
7. Stevia extract, to taste
8. 10 g almonds

Instructions:

1. In a large pan, add the pumpkin pieces, stevia extract, and a cup of water.
2. Cover the pan and cook the pumpkin on medium heat for 24 to 30 minutes.
3. In a small bowl, dissolve corn flour with milk until smooth.
4. Once the pumpkin is cooked, add the dissolved cornflour and mix. Cook until the liquid thickens.
5. Sprinkle cinnamon and desiccated coconut then mix.
6. Transfer to a serving dish. Sprinkle almonds and pomegranate pearls before serving.

Grilled Vermouth Tuna

Ingredients:

- 2 tbsp. dry vermouth
- 1 tbsp. olive oil
- 2 tbsp. fresh basil, minced
- 2 green onions, chopped
- 1 clove garlic, minced
- 1/2 tsp. dried marjoram
- 1/4 tsp. red flakes of pepper
- 1 lb. tuna steak, cut 3/4- to 1-inch thick
- 1 lemon

Instructions:

1. Combine all the vermouth, olive oil, onion, and spices. Pour the mixture over the tuna and marinate in the fridge for 1 to 2 hours.

2. Preheat the broiler or charcoal grill. Spray the broiler pan with non-stick cooking spray.
3. Cover the fish and charcoal grill over medium coals or broil it about six inches from the heat source for 4 minutes per side or until the fish turns firm and opaque.
4. Baste the fish with the marinade two times while cooking.
5. Cut the lemon into wedges and serve the fish fresh from the grill with lemon wedges on the side.

Oatmeal Yogurt Smoothie

Ingredients:

- 1/2 cup rolled oats
- 1 cup almond milk
- 1/3 cup plain yogurt
- 1 banana, sliced
- 1/4 cup strawberries, raspberries, or blackberries

Instructions:

1. Combine the oats, yogurt, and 3/4 cup almond milk in a bowl. Cover and refrigerate overnight. Set aside 1/4 cup for later, to be added to the blender in the morning.
2. After refrigerating overnight, pour the mixture into a blender and add the remaining 1/4 cup of almond milk. Add more if it is still too thick.
3. Add the banana and berries then blend until it turns smooth.
4. Serve immediately.

Oven-Baked Salmon with Radish

Ingredients:

- 2 medium onions, sliced half-inch thick
- 4 tbsp. extra-virgin olive oil, divided
- 2 lemons zest
- 1 tsp. kosher salt, divided
- 4 5-oz. skin-on salmon fillets
- 6 large radishes, cut in wedges, with some thinly sliced to be used for garnish
- 1 1/2 tsp. cracked black pepper
- 1 tsp. Old Bay seasoning
- 1/2 tsp. sugar
- for garnish: flaky sea salt, fresh cilantro

Instructions:

1. Preheat your oven to 325°F.
2. Place a large cast-iron skillet. Set heat to high.
3. Cook onions, pressing them down occasionally for 10 to 15 minutes or until one side is completely charred.
4. Repeat the process for 8 to 10 minutes more to char the other side.
5. Transfer to a bowl and cover tightly to steam for 15 minutes.
6. In another bowl, mix 2 tbsp. of oil, pepper, lemon zest, and 1/2 tsp. salt.
7. In the same skillet where you cooked the onions, over medium heat, add 1 tbsp. oil to heat.

8. Place the salmon skin-side down first. Spoon lemon zest mixture and spread over the salmon.
9. Put the skillet in the oven and bake for 14 to 16 minutes or until cooked through.
10. In a saucepan, bring a small amount of water to a boil. Blanched the radish for 5 to 6 minutes until tender. Drain and pat dry.
11. Dry the saucepan and add the remaining tbsp. of oil, and old bay seasoning. Bring to sizzle for 1 minute over medium heat.
12. Remove from heat and stir in the radish. Cover and keep warm.
13. Combine the onion with the remaining 1/2 tsp. salt and sugar and using a food processor puree until smooth.
14. Pour the puree over the salmon and radish before serving. Garnish with cilantro, flaky salt, and sliced radish if you desire.

Pesto Chicken Cauliflower Pizza and Salad Mix

Ingredients:

Roasted Chicken:

- 5 boneless, skinless chicken thighs (about 1-1/4 lb.), trimmed
- 1/2 tsp. ground pepper
- 1/4 tsp. salt

Pizza:

- 1 (7 to 12-ounce) cauliflower pizza crust (frozen)

- 1/4 cup prepared pesto
- 1 cup part-skim mozzarella cheese, shredded

Salad:

- 1 chopped small head of iceberg lettuce
- 1 cup finely chopped cauliflower
- 1 cup halved cherry tomatoes
- 4 jarred pepperoncini, sliced
- 1/4 cup chopped pepperoni (1 ounce)

Italian Dressing:

- 3/4 cup red-wine vinegar
- 5 tbsp. water
- 1 1/2 tbsp. sugar
- 1 tbsp. Dijon mustard
- 1 large clove of garlic
- 2 tsp. dried basil
- 2 tsp. dried oregano
- 1/2 tsp. salt
- 1/2 tsp. ground pepper
- 1 3/4 cups extra-virgin olive oil

Instructions:

1. Set the oven at 425°F to preheat.
2. Place the chicken on a baking dish. Sprinkle it with salt and pepper.

3. Bake it for 14 to 16 minutes or until the temperature inside the chicken reaches 165°F.
4. Shred 1 chicken thigh. Store the other 4 chicken thighs for another use.
5. For the cauliflower pizza crust, spread the pesto over the crust.
6. Sprinkle it with mozzarella and the shredded chicken thigh. Bake according to package instructions.
7. Prepare salad dressing by combining water, sugar, vinegar, mustard, garlic, oregano, basil, salt, and pepper in a blender.
8. Puree the mixture until it turns smooth. Slowly add oil over the puree while the blender is still running. Turn off when the puree turns creamy. Keep half of the dressing for another use.
9. Prepare the salad mix by combining all the salad ingredients in a large serving bowl. Toss the salad with the dressing just before serving.
10. Cut a slice of pizza and serve it with the salad.

Conclusion

Congratulations on taking the steps to understand more about osteoporosis and its associated diet! Osteoporosis is a condition that affects both men and women and can be very serious. It is caused by a decrease in bone density, resulting in bones becoming fragile and easily broken. An osteoporosis diet is an important part of treating the condition and has been found to help reduce the rate of bone loss.

The key components of an osteoporosis diet include lots of calcium, vitamin D, magnesium, zinc, potassium, phosphorus, protein, boron, and selenium. Eating foods that are high in these ingredients can help to increase your bone mineral density significantly. It is also important to limit sodium intake as this can leach calcium from your bones resulting in further weakening them. Drinking plenty of water is essential for hydration which helps to prevent further deterioration.

It is also important to get regular physical activity as exercise helps strengthen bones and muscles. Weight-bearing exercises such as walking, running, or stair climbing are particularly beneficial for those with low bone density. Even simple activities such as gardening can have a positive effect on overall muscle health by increasing strength.

Finally, it's essential to have a balanced diet that includes all the major food groups—fruit & vegetables; whole grains; proteins; dairy & dairy alternatives; wealthy fats; and healthy proteins like beans & nuts are all great sources of vital nutrients for bone health. Paying attention to what you eat each day will help you remain healthy while optimizing your bone mass so you don't suffer from complications due to osteoporosis down the road! With the right diet plan and regular physical activity, you can achieve optimal protection against this disease which often goes unnoticed until it's too late.

References

7-day osteoporosis diet plan. (2017, January 25). Healthline. https://www.healthline.com/health/managing-osteoporosis/7-day-osteoporosis-diet-plan.

Australia, H. (2023, March 23). Osteoporosis [Http://purl.org/ontology/nhccn#text_html]. https://www.healthdirect.gov.au/osteoporosis.

Boston, 677 Huntington Avenue & Ma 02115 +1495-1000. (2012, September 18). Vitamin d. The Nutrition Source. https://www.hsph.harvard.edu/nutritionsource/vitamin-d/.

Dental health and osteoporosis—Humana. (n.d.). Retrieved April 1, 2023, from https://www.humana.com/dental-insurance/dental-resources/osteoporosis-dental.

How much sodium should I eat per day? (n.d.). Www.Heart.Org. Retrieved April 1, 2023, from https://www.heart.org/en/healthy-living/healthy-eating/eat-smart/sodium/how-much-sodium-should-i-eat-per-day.

Osteoporosis diet & nutrition: Foods for bone health. (n.d.). Bone Health & Osteoporosis Foundation. Retrieved April 1,

2023, from https://www.bonehealthandosteoporosis.org/patients/treatment/nutrition/.

Osteoporosis: Symptoms, causes, tests & treatment. (n.d.). Cleveland Clinic. Retrieved April 1, 2023, from https://my.clevelandclinic.org/health/diseases/4443-osteoporosis.

Services, D. of H. & H. (n.d.). Menopause and osteoporosis. Retrieved April 1, 2023, from http://www.betterhealth.vic.gov.au/health/conditionsandtreatments/menopause-and-osteoporosis.

Should you be taking a calcium supplement? (n.d.). Retrieved April 1, 2023, from https://www.houstonmethodist.org/blog/articles/2021/oct/calcium-supplements-how-much-calcium-is-too-much/.

www.ingramcontent.com/pod-product-compliance
Ingram Content Group UK Ltd.
Pitfield, Milton Keynes, MK11 3LW, UK
UKHW021353221025
8529UKWH00034B/659